Integrated Yoga

of related interest

Yoga for Children with Autism Spectrum Disorders
A Step-by-Step Guide for Parents and Caregivers
Dion E. Betts and Stacey W. Betts
Forewords by Louise Goldberg and Joshua S. Betts
ISBN 978 1 84310 817 7

Tai Chi Chuan and the Code of Life
Revealing the Deeper Mysteries of China's Ancient Art for Health and Harmony
Graham Horwood
ISBN 978 1 84310 580 0

Vital Breath of the Dao
Chinese Shamanic Tiger Qigong – Laohu Gong
Master Zhongxian Wu
ISBN 978 1 84310 579 4

Understanding Sensory Dysfunction
Learning, Development and Sensory Dysfunction in Autism Spectrum Disorders, ADHD, Learning Disabilities and Bipolar Disorder
Polly Godwin Emmons and Liz McKendry Anderson
ISBN 978 1 84310 806 1

Sensory Smarts
A Book for Kids with ADHD or Autism Spectrum Disorders Struggling with Sensory Integration Problems
Kathleen A. Chara and Paul J. Chara, Jr.
With Christian P. Chara
Illustrated by J.M. Berns
ISBN 978 1 84310 783 5

Sensory Perceptual Issues in Autism and Asperger Syndrome
Different Sensory Experiences – Different Perceptual Worlds
Olga Bogdashina
Forewords by Wendy Lawson and Theo Peeters
ISBN 978 1 84310 166 6

Kids in the Syndrome Mix of ADHD, LD, Asperger's, Tourette's, Bipolar, and More!
The one stop guide for parents, teachers, and other professionals
Martin L. Kutscher MD, with contributions from Tony Attwood PhD and Robert R. Wolff MD
ISBN 978 1 84310 811 5

The Verbal Behavior Approach
How to Teach Children with Autism and Related Disorders
Mary Lynch Barbera with Tracy Rasmussen
Foreword by Mark L. Sundberg, Ph.D., BCBA
ISBN 978 1 84310 852 8

Integrated Yoga

Yoga with a Sensory Integrative Approach

Nicole Cuomo

Jessica Kingsley Publishers
London and Philadelphia

First published in 2007
by Jessica Kingsley Publishers
116 Pentonville Road
London N1 9JB, UK
and
400 Market Street, Suite 400
Philadelphia, PA 19106, USA

www.jkp.com

Disclaimer
The author of this material is not liable or responsible to any person for any damage caused or alleged to be caused directly or indirectly by the information contained in this book.

Library of Congress Cataloging in Publication Data

Cuomo, Nicole C., 1965-
 Integrated yoga : yoga with a sensory integrative approach / Nicole Cuomo.
   p. cm.
 ISBN-13: 978-1-84310-862-7 (pb)
 ISBN-10: 1-84310-862-3 (pb)
 1. Hatha yoga for children. 2. Sensorimotor integration. I. Title.
 RJ133.7.C86 2007
 613.7'046083--dc22

                        2006101869

British Library Cataloguing in Publication Data
A CIP catalogue record for this book is available from the British Library

ISBN 978 1 84310 862 7

Printed and bound in the United States by
Thomson-Shore, Inc.

Contents

Acknowledgements

I would like to thank my husband Doug, my son Neal, and friends, family, and students for the encouragement and support during my long years of education and practice. My thanks also to the children I have worked with over the last 15 years for their great ideas. Finally, I would especially like to thank my niece, Erica R. Buehler, for posing for the photographs in this book.

Introduction

The idea for *Integrated Yoga* came to me after years of practice as an occupational therapist and yoga practitioner. I have worked with a variety of children and adults with different sensory systems and through this came to understand that my own sensory system fluctuated and that I needed to vary my yoga practice in order to stay focused and present. There are so many wonderful books on both yoga and sensory integration it just did not make sense to reinvent the wheel, so this book gives a brief introduction to both topics and, importantly, how they are complementary to each other. I offer suggestions for practice with children and these concepts can also be adapted for use with adults.

This book is not intended to be a sensory integration treatment book, that takes the place of working with a qualified professional therapist, but rather as an enhancement to treatment. As all therapists and parents know there is no cookbook for working with children, only guidelines that have to be tweaked so that the fit is perfect.

Approach the subject with an open heart and an open mind, and don't forget to breathe.

Peace, Nicole

1 What is Yoga?

Yoga has been practiced for thousands of years. Yoga is a Sanskrit word meaning to "yoke up" or unite. A number of books have been written on different kinds of yoga, from ancient texts to modern interpretation practices. My intention here is to provide a brief introduction to a very deep practice.

Yoga is the union of body, mind, and spirit. The practice of yoga should be done with an open heart and mind. It can allow you to move towards new ways of balance, serenity, and freedom – physically and emotionally. Many people practice yoga to center themselves and to relax from a hectic lifestyle.

Hatha Yoga is the type of yoga that focuses on physical movements, called *asanas* (postures). This includes movement, breathing, and stretching. This is typically what you do when you go to a yoga class.

Raja Yoga is mind yoga; this practice is more devotional and includes meditation and prayer, allowing one to become a free being. This is generally the type of yoga one moves towards after practicing hatha yoga.

Pranayama is breath control or controlled breathing. By controlling the breath you can control the mind. If you notice your breathing when you are stressed you will note that you often hold your breath and/or breathe rapidly in short breaths. When relaxed you take longer, fuller, easier, and more rhythmical breaths.

Whatever type of yoga you practice it can allow you to slow down, relax, and feel present and aware.

2 Sensory Integration – A Brief Overview

The theory of sensory integration, also called "SI", is a process of neural organization that allows us to function within our different environments. Jean Ayres, the founder of this theory, surmised that our brains receive sensory information from the sensory receptors in our bodies; this information is directed to the brain where it is organized and interpreted and the brain then responds with something called "an adaptive response". For example, if I bumped my leg on a table I would most likely drop down and hold onto the area that hurt in order to relieve the pain and to protect it from further damage.

The primary sensory systems in the theory of SI are the tactile, vestibular, and proprioceptive senses. These are sensory systems that we are not all necessarily familiar with.

The *tactile system* is the one we are most aware of. The receptors for this lie in our skin and give us information regarding texture, temperature, shape, and size. This sense allows us to discriminate – "is it scratchy or soft?" – and also serves as a protective response – "there is a very scary spider climbing up my arm, I need to react".

The vestibular system is located within the inner ear. It gives us information on where we are in relation to gravity. It allows us to make adjustments in the body if we happen to fall forward or lose balance in any direction.

The proprioceptive system has receptors located in the muscles and joints. This gives information regarding body position and resistance. For example, I can walk without looking at my legs and feet. My sense of proprioception allows me to move and make any adjustments without using my vision. It also helps make adjustments when lifting an object, depending on whether it is heavy or light.

The visual, auditory, gustatory, touch, and taste senses are also important in this theory and may be accessed during treatment to provide an adaptive response.

Sometimes there is misunderstanding in our sensory processing

We all have our own individual and unique sensory systems; while some of us may prefer bland foods, others crave foods that are spicy. Our differences in sensory situations are based upon how we respond to different sensory input. People with a well-integrated vestibular system will be drawn towards activities that challenge them, while those who have systems not as well integrated may be drawn towards more passive activities.

Some adults and children can set up their living situations so that they are nurturing their sensory systems and can therefore function effectively within their environment. This may not be possible for other children and adults, and consequently they may have great difficulty functioning in a world that feels out of control. This is the reason that some people choose to operate jack hammers, while others choose to work in a library.

The threshold idea

There is a theory that postulates that sensory input is recognized as a threshold response. We all have different threshold levels. For example, I may need more movement input in the form of jumping or spinning before I begin to feel dizzy, whereas a friend may spin around once and feel uncomfortably giddy. This idea transfers to all levels of sensory input and can explain why some people like the television volume turned up high, others will cover their ears if it is too loud. Some like wearing only soft clothing, while others can be comfortable wearing any texture.

Children and adults who have difficulty with sensory processing may have a sensitivity in a specific area, such as with tactile input (i.e. dislikes being touched, will only wear certain clothing, may fear haircuts, etc.). These sensitivities can also be seen in the areas of taste and smell (gagging at typical foods), vestibular perception (easily sick, or anxious when on a surface or in an object that is moving), auditory perception (will become upset/scared with noises such as a vacuum cleaner, blender, or loud TV), and visual perception (can become easily over-whelmed in busy places such as a mall). This can be described as having a low threshold for sensory input, meaning that the threshold for "typical" sensory input (that which is easily tolerated by some), is overwhelming.

A child or adult with a high threshold for sensory input will get the sensory input that those around them do, but may not register it. For example, someone who requires intense vestibular input to be aware of gravity can be seen in constant movement, wriggling in chairs, flying across the playground, etc. If there are problems in the proprioceptive and tactile areas there is usually difficulty in grading movements, and the problems that can be seen are breaking toys from rough play, squeezing toys, and fingering foods to the point of mashing them.

Some children and adults can have both sensitivities and sensory-seeking sensory systems. There can be a mix of high and low thresholds depending on the type of input. The ability to integrate the senses allows us to perform complex functions in our environments; for children this could be performing in school and playing with friends.

With adults it could be being able to function at work, complete all the necessary household chores, and being able to work well with others.

Here is a brief overview of some of the things that you may see when working with people with sensory processing problems.

Tactile

Under-responsive:

- may get injured and not realize
- may have poor body awareness
- may drop items and not realize
- often compensate with visual skills.

Over-responsive:

- overly sensitive to being touched
- may react aggressively to being touched
- often dislike others being in close proximity
- may be choosy about clothing and/or foods
- may always choose to wear long-sleeve shirts.

Proprioception

- often have stiff uncoordinated movements
- often have difficulty grading movements
- frequently fall
- unable to do things without looking.

Vestibular

Under-responsive:

- tend to crave movement, often in motion, and like to move quickly

- often have difficulty sitting still

- usually have low muscle tone, particularly in the extensors

- tend to have poor endurance.

Over-responsive:

- intolerant of movement (may be fearful or aggressive)

- may experience motion sickness

- do not like physical play, such as roughhousing

- dislikes or avoids physical play (playgrounds)

- uncomfortable when feet are off the ground.

This is a complicated system and theory and the effects are many. There are numerous books and articles that explain the theory in detail; if you wish to explore the topic further refer to the suggested reading list (see p.97).

3 How do Yoga and Sensory Integration Work Together?

Hatha yoga is the practice of movement, breathing (called *pranayama*), and focus. As an occupational therapist and yoga teacher, I have found that on some days I need a more vigorous practice and on others a more relaxing practice, in order to be present and set myself up for the day. I have also found in teaching yoga that some people prefer a more vigorous practice – using a flowing sequence of challenging postures, while others prefer a slow practice that focuses more on maintaining the poses, on *pranayama* and ending with a long relaxing period (called *savasana*) in order to feel fulfilled.

When one is involved and participating in yoga it is called a practice. The reason it is called this is because the repetition of postures, refocusing on the breath and movement, and relaxing, is a practice which must be sustained in order to be effective. If you decide to do yoga once in a while, it can have immediate benefits. However, when you decide to follow the path of practice it is a daily (or at least weekly) ritual which constantly brings you back into a state of awareness. This awareness has long-term benefits, allowing you to function more proficiently within your daily activities with clarity of mind and body.

Yoga with children is approached differently than it is for adults. Kids usually like to move; moving enables them to explore their environment and master basic developmental skills. Kids also don't want a detailed explanation for each posture and how it will benefit them. They want yoga to be fun, and will participate if they enjoy it and if they feel good after practicing. When using yoga with children we can set them up for a lifetime of clarity and focus, which can help them to overcome the inevitable difficulties and obstacles in life. This is especially true for children (and indeed adults) with sensory processing difficulties, as they are often misunderstood by the general population.

Children and adults often seek out professional assistance in overcoming sensory processing difficulties, by working with therapists trained in sensory integration treatment. The suggested activities are not a substitute for professional treatment, but rather an enhancement to professional treatment, that can be done in the clinic, in the classroom, and at home.

Yoga combines movement with weight-bearing positions. Weight bearing on joints helps to improve stability and promotes body awareness. For those with anxiety or frustration, yoga allows an opportunity to slow down, focus on movement and breathing, and become more centered. When practicing barefoot, your feet have tactile input; this can help with discrimination and can also help children who have poor body-in-space understanding. Moving in and out of a yoga pose involves motor planning; sequential and fluid movements are experienced. Sometimes, kids with sensory problems just try to get through an activity without really understanding how to move their bodies; yoga provides an opportunity for self-discovery.

It is important to remember that there is no cookbook recipe for treating and working with those who have sensory processing difficulties. There are general guidelines which must be constantly re-evaluated for effectiveness. I believe that by having a yoga practice and allowing yourself to be focused, calm, and present, you can expand your observational skills and guide those around you who may have sensory difficulties. As one of my students said to me years ago, "sometimes I just gotta move".

4 Yoga Practice and Age Groups

How to do yoga

- It is best to use a nonskid sticky mat; you can also use a rug, or towel (if on a carpet) or other nonskid surface.

- No shoes – it is best to do yoga in bare feet, however some children will not want to remove their socks and that's okay too. (You may have to work up to barefeet.)

- Music – which can be lively or relaxing. (For more detail see Chapter 5.)

- Set aside specific times throughout the day to practice. These times could vary and could incorporate one to two poses or more.

- Don't practice after a full meal, wait two hours. It's best to practice on an empty stomach, but after a small snack is fine.

Age groups: general guidelines

- *Preschool – ages 3–5 years:* Children are learning to use space, and having fun moving around. Children discover space through play and like to use whole body movements, and imaginative play. Don't do too many jumping transitions as this can overtax cartilage and bone structure.

- *Kindergarten–2nd grade – ages 5–8 years:* Kids gain more motor control and are stronger, they can be tireless and tend to learn quicker. It can be hard for them to know when to stop, particularly if they become overexcited. Try to keep them from overstretching; you can use imagination and stories to develop postures.

- *3rd–5th grade – ages 8–11 years:* Kids begin to like challenges rather than fantasy and stories. This is a good age to begin to learn technique. Kids this age tend to like rules and games with rules. Remind them that yoga is not competitive, but cooperative.

These age guidelines are just that: guidelines. Use your own discretion as children have different abilities and some will attempt and enjoy activities in any and all age ranges. Have fun, experiment, and play.

Older children can help lead younger children and may be great inspirations for creative stories (as long as they are not too scary). It is important to offer encouragement and praise. Remember that yoga with kids is different than it is for adults. Yoga with kids should focus more on exploration and less on alignment; however do be cautious of patterns that may cause injury. One thing I have found is that kids like to put their heads down and weight bear on their necks, which can cause injury. Use your eyes and your heart to guide you. If you are unsure whether or not something could be potentially dangerous, it is best to move on to another posture. Better to be safe than to be sorry.

Some final key thoughts to consider include: if kids appear to be getting overstimulated with movement or when tipping their heads, follow with a pose that offers full body input in weight bearing (such as plank pose); or rest in relaxation pose and encourage slow breathing. If kids appear to be getting drowsy, use more movement to "wake" them up.

5　Integration of the Practices

It is important to be aware of developmental levels when working with children and yoga. Things that may be challenging and fun for a three-year-old might be boring for a nine-year-old. The postures can be used in a sequence and individually. Coming up with stories or having kids make up their own while practicing can go a long way to increase the fun and creativity.

Using music during the practice can reap wonderful results; however, be selective in the type of music you choose. If you are looking for calming activities for a child with sensitivities, use beats that are slow and rhythmical. The music can be slow chants or classical music; drumming music tends to be very grounding. You may have to experiment to be sure you are using effective music. If you are looking to provide a great amount of input for a child that appears sluggish and tired, music with changing tempos and alternating rhythms works well. I have found that when using quick tempo music like that of the Beach Boys or similar, you must be cognizant of providing the sensory input without overstimulating the child (or the adults for that matter). Often times the first session with music may not go as smoothly as you would like, as kids can be overattentive to the music and not the activity, however the novelty usually wears off and the music is an added enhancement.

Different ways to use the poses

You can set up sessions to focus on one or two poses with a follow-up activity, or you can sequence several of them together and do a follow-up activity on one pose. I strongly suggest you go through all of the poses individually prior to attempting the sun or moon salute. Begin each session with a breathing exercise, depending on whether or not the children need to be calmed or alerted. Once the breathing is completed move on to the physical poses. Use one or many, depending on the time, space available, and size of the group. If you are working one-on-one let the child choose one pose and you choose the next. You can make a card for each pose and have the kids pull a card out of the deck and sequence the poses that way. Drawing, painting, and coloring are great expressive activities to incorporate into the yoga practice. Kids can draw, color, or paint their favorite pose. Remember above all, this should be fun and build the child's confidence and help them to be calmed or alerted.

6 Basic Postures

This chapter is divided into three sections: breathing, postures, and sequences. Each pose is described in detail, and its benefits explained. Follow-up activities are suggested by age, and methods of dealing with any sensory problems that a child might have are described.

Breathing practice

Most yogic breathing is through the nose. However, some children may not understand the concept (or may have stuffy noses). If you are trying to teach breathing through the nose and it is not working, try breathing in through the nose and blowing out through the lips. Alternatively, mouth breathing can be slowed so that the child is breathing deeply. Demonstrate the options.

When performing breathing exercises in the sitting position it is important to keep a tall straight back, with the head held up. This allows the rib cage and diaphragm to rise and fall with the inhalations and exhalations. For those with poor posture, some of the breathing can be done while lying on the back. You can also have kids sit up against a wall for back support. If a child is asthmatic, breathing should be slow and steady; a physician's clearance should be sought prior to participation.

Belly breathing*

This is a good way to start and end a practice session. It allows the focus to be on the breath. Hands are placed on the belly, eyes closed. Encourage the child to feel the breath making their belly go up and down. Breath is slow and regulated. This breath is appropriate for all age groups.

Belly breathing has a relaxing effect and can be done standing, sitting or lying on the back once it is learned.

---

*   Some children with sensory sensitivities may have paradoxical breathing – this is when the diaphragm raises up instead of down on the inhale. Keep using belly breathing to teach correct breathing. If there is no change I suggest that the child work with a therapist trained in manual therapy in order to release restrictions in the diaphragm and rib cage.

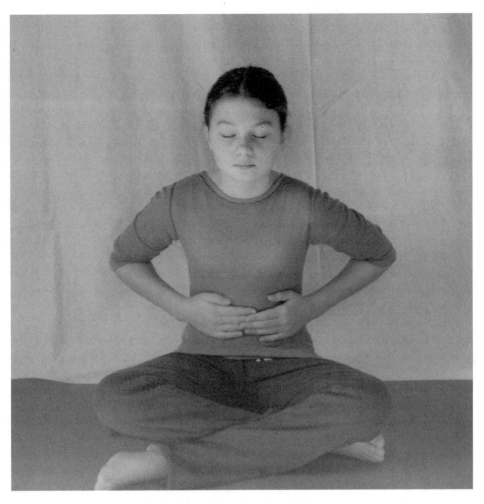

Belly breathing

Breath of fire

Performed in a cross-legged, sitting position with the hands placed on the knees, eyes closed. A quick inhale and exhale (forced inhale and exhale) through the nose. The belly should move in and out quickly. Begin with five repetitions followed by a slow, deep breath. Continue again with five and increase the number of repetitions as the practice becomes easier.

This breath can be used for ages 5–8 and 8–11; younger children may become overexcited. It is best to use this with kids who have under-responsive systems, as those with sensitivities may easily become over-stimulated. If it appears as though kids are getting a little too hyper, return to belly breathing while lying down. Children with sensitivities may find this breathing to be too alerting and may cause distress. Some kids and adults get dizzy when performing the breath of fire. It should be performed for only five repetitions at most when beginning. Asthmatic children should not do the breath of fire.

The breath of fire is an alerting technique. It is meant to alert and awaken.

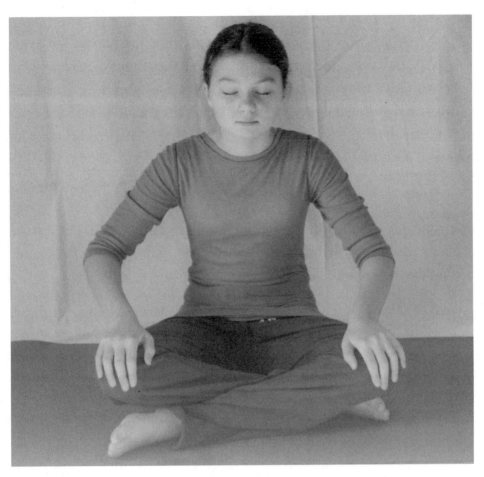

Breath of fire

Alternate nostril breathing

This breath is known as a nerve cleanser. The child should sit cross-legged. Hold the right hand with the index and middle finger held down into the palm (this is known as *mirgi mudra*, "deer head" position). Bring the right hand up to the face, placing the thumb beside the right nostril and the ring finger and pinky by the left nostril. Breathe out completely. Close the right nostril with the thumb and breathe in through the left nostril. Close the left nostril with the pinky and ring finger and exhale through the right nostril. Inhale through the right nostril, close the right nostril with the thumb and exhale through the left nostril. That is one round. Close the right nostril and continue as before. Complete 6–8 rounds.

- Best used with kids aged 5–8 and 8–11 years. Younger children may need more guidance with the hand position and assistance for left/right discrimination.

This breath is good for all sensory systems as it has a centering effect. It is also good for children who have mucus and phlegm problems (keep tissues handy).

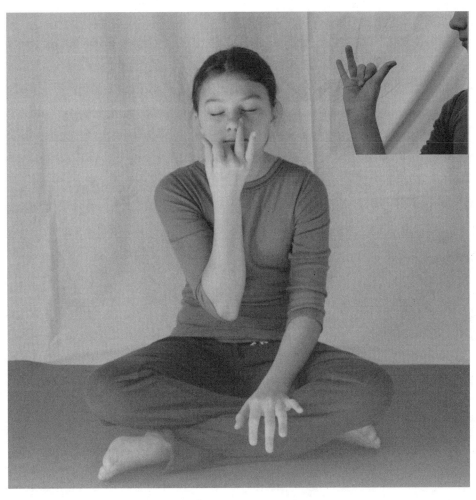

Alternate nostril breathing

Langhana

A breathing practice which emphasizes the exhale. Breathe in for a count of 4–5 and breathe out for a count of 6–7. The extension of the exhale causes an autonomic nervous system response which promotes relaxation. This is a great breathing exercise to practice if children appear anxious. Langhana can be done sitting or lying on the back. This can be used for all ages, provided the child can count or, at least, has an understanding of what numbers are. Demonstration and verbal cueing throughout is recommended.

This breathing practice is an excellent tool for children with sensitivities as it encourages relaxation, which is often lacking in their world.

The physical postures (*asanas*)
Mountain

All standing poses begin and end in mountain pose. Stand with feet slightly apart or together. Equal weight is on both feet, legs straight, with body extending up towards the clouds. Arms are resting at the sides of the body and the head and neck are in alignment. You can encourage kids to look at something on a wall in front of them to keep their gaze up.

- *3–5-year-olds:* You could use a slow gentle song that is familiar to them while they hold the posture. Alternatively the kids can slowly march, gently stomping their feet, then stop in mountain pose to really feel the body position. Another idea is to say the ABC song, or count to five or ten while holding the pose.

- *5–8-year-olds:* The children can practice belly breathing while in the pose or count even or odd numbers. They can also march – emphasize slow then fast stomping for increased sensory input.

- *8–11-year-olds:* They can perform belly breathing, the breath of fire, and alternate nostril breathing. They can also hold the pose in silence focusing on their own breath.

This pose develops stability and balance and promotes centering.

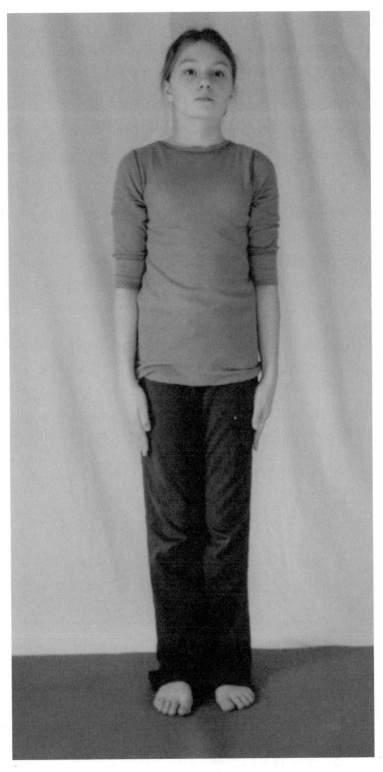

Mountain

Straight tree

Start in mountain pose. Inhale and raise the arms up over the head lifting up onto the toes at the same time. Breathe out and lower heels and arms. Repeat.

- *3–5-year-olds:* Have the kids stretch upwards as if they are growing like trees or flowers. As a complementary activity, plant seeds with the kids or have them color pictures of trees and flowers.

- *5–8-year-olds:* Begin emphasizing balance and strength. Pair the practice with a science activity or with leaf rubbings. Explore types of trees – bent trees and straight trees. This would be a good time to plant vegetables or saplings with the children to show them how things grow up towards the sun.

- *8–11-year-olds:* As with the younger age group, emphasize balance and strength. Begin encouraging the kids to hold their posture in the balance, starting with a few seconds and working up to more time. Older kids can practice gently moving back and forth as if blowing in the wind.

Practicing this pose brings calmness, balance, and strength.

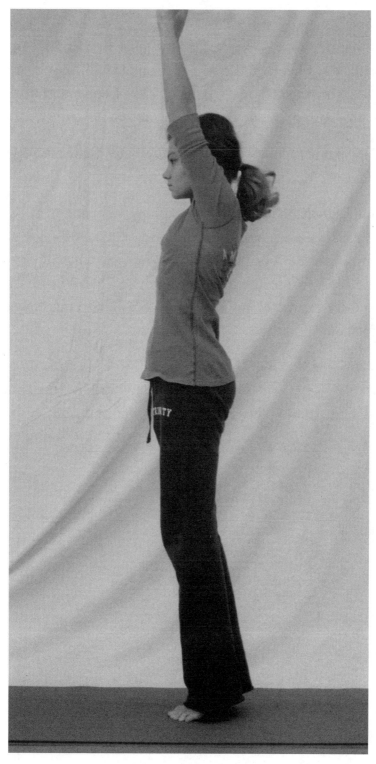

Straight tree

Side stretch

Start in mountain pose. Raise the left arm above the head, alongside the ear, keep the right hand on the side of the thigh. Inhale and stretch the left arm up to the sky and on the exhale tilt the trunk and slide the right hand down the thigh while bringing the raised hand over the head.

- *3–5-year-olds:* Switch sides and alternate. Make sure they don't move too quickly but gently feel the stretch.

- *5–8-year-olds:* The children should move in and out of the posture. Start a discussion about the body and the rib cage. Use anatomy charts designed for kids to show them where the ribs begin and end. Use imaginative descriptions such as "the rib cage protects the heart and lungs, it is like a castle", so that they can understand.

- *8–11-year-olds:* Kids hold the pose – to each side – for several seconds. This would be a good time to introduce the children to basic anatomy – the skeleton, the spine, and rib cage.

The children will stretch both sides of their bodies.

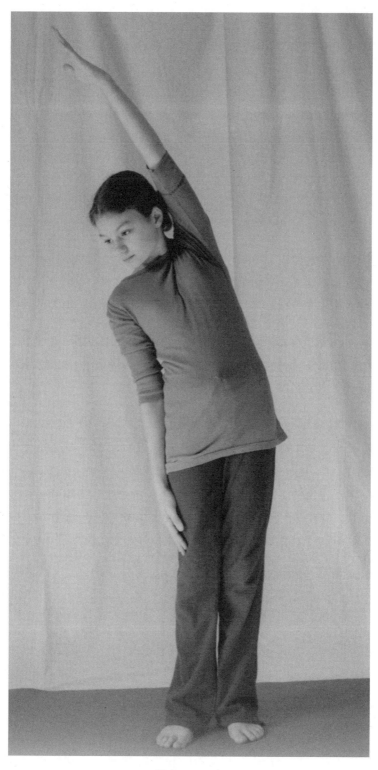

Side stretch

Fold in half

Start in mountain pose. Breathe in and raise the arms up over the head. Breathe out and bend forward at the hips, pointing the fingers towards the toes. Inhale and return to mountain pose. Repeat. (When staying in the fold pose, either wrap the hands around the calves – which some find more comfortable – or keep the hands out in front.)

- *3–5-year-olds:* You can sing "this is the way we bend in half, bend in half, bend in half, this is the way we bend in half so early in the morning" while they practice.

- *5–8-year-olds:* The children should move in and out of the posture. Start a discussion about things that bend and things that you don't bend; this can include body parts and objects.

- *8–11-year-olds:* Have the children move in and out of the posture, then have them stay bent forward, allowing the stretch to open up the back of the body.

Kids with vestibular sensitivity may not want to bend all the way forward. Let them move forward into a comfortable range, and come back slowly and gently. Allow them to repeat. Over time you will be able to work the child into the more forward posture. You can also modify the pose by having them bend over a desk or table, or have them reach out to a wall in front of them while they gently bend forward.

The fold in half stretches and strengthens the spine.

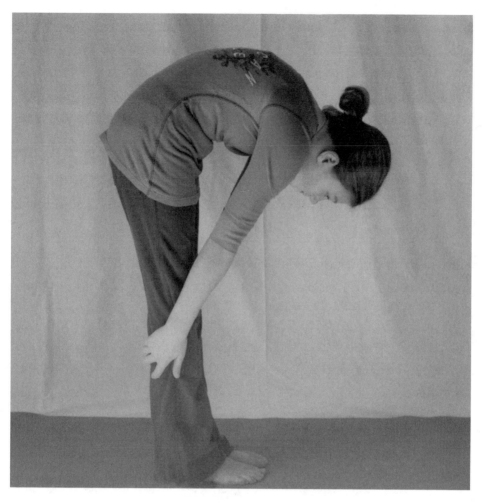

Fold in half

Chair and chair twist

Begin in mountain pose. Breathe in and raise the arms over the head. Exhale and bring the arms straight out in front, while lowering as if to sit on a chair. Move in and out of the posture with the breath, then stay and breathe out while twisting the shoulders to the side, rotating or twisting at the trunk, and bringing the back of the arm to the outside of the leg. The twist should be done on the exhale. Inhale to straighten, and come back to chair. Come to standing and repeat, twisting to the other side.

- *5–8 years olds:* Have the children move in and out of the posture, then stay briefly. If the children look well-balanced you can have them try the twist. Have the kids cut out different chairs from furniture catalogs and ask them to describe what they like about them, why do they think it would be comfortable? Gather fabric samples and let them feel and discuss different textures.

- *8–11-year-olds:* The kids can move in and out and attempt the twist. Have the children design their own chairs, describing or drawing what they would be made of, how big, etc., and why.

Kids with vestibular difficulties may not want to try the twist. That's okay, keep working on the chair pose without the twist and gradually build up their strength and balance.

For kids with vestibular sensitivities and balance issues move slowly and deliberately through the pose (in and out), to challenge their balance and improve strength.

Encourage children who are under-responsive to move in and out quickly before staying in the pose, to build strength.

For children with tactile sensitivities it is a good opportunity to let them feel different textures. Often a child who is sensitive to touch will be more comfortable if they can initiate the touch. Put fabric samples down in the middle of a circle of children and let them explore. Once the kids are comfortable with the textures in their hands you can ask them to rub the fabrics on their arms and feet.

This pose helps develop thighs and knees, and works on balance and trunk rotation.

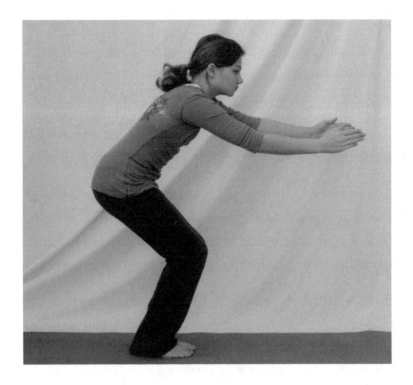

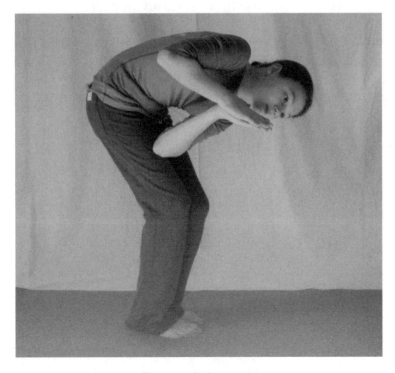

Chair and chair twist

Warrior 1

Start in mountain pose. Step the left foot forward (the right foot may turn out slightly), inhale and raise both arms over the head. Exhale and bend the left knee. Move in and out of pose, then switch sides.

- *3–5-year-olds:* As kids go into the posture and stay, have them say a mantra such as "I am a hero, I am cool, and I am strong".

- *5–8-year-olds:* Allow the kids to move in and out of the posture, then stay. Include discussion on what a warrior is, keep positive thoughts and words on the agenda. Include mantras such as "I am strong, I am peaceful, and I can make a difference".

- *8–11-year-olds:* Have the children stay in the posture for longer periods and focus on deep breathing. They can make up a story cooperatively while in the posture. Start them off by saying "there was a warrior at my house and she/he was… and have the kids add one fact each then switch sides in the pose and continue the story, keeping the tone and content positive.

For a calming effect encourage the children to speak slowly and quietly. For an excitatory response have them shout louder.

Children benefit from this exercise as it develops strength and determination.

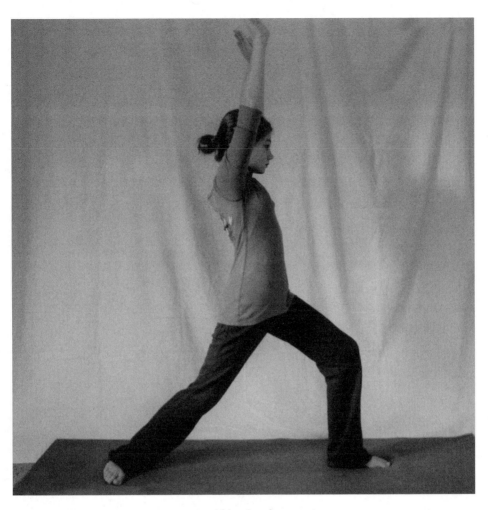

Warrior 1

Warrior 2

Start in mountain pose. Step the left foot forward and turn the right foot
out slightly (about 45–90 degrees). Inhale and raise the arms to
shoulder level – the left arm in front of the body, the right arm behind.
Exhale and lower down by bending the front knee. Switch sides.

For guidance on the various age groups see warrior 1 p.40. For a
calming effect use mantras and stories slowly spoken, for an excitatory
response use loud mantras. This practice promotes the development of
strength and determination.

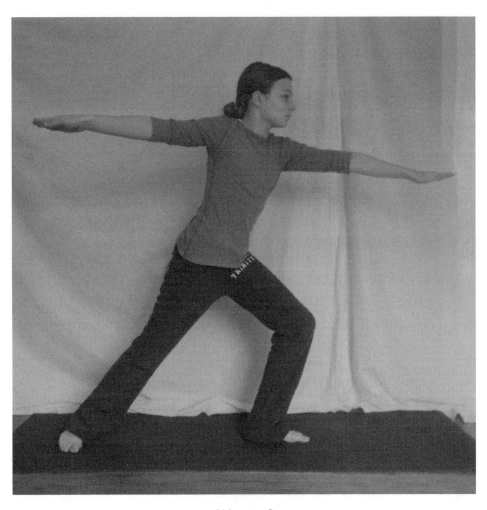

Warrior 2

Warrior stretch

From the warrior 2 finishing position, bend at the trunk (a lateral bend of the body) to lower the front arm onto the thigh. The other arm reaches straight up, and over the head.

- *3–5-year-olds:* Have the kids go into the posture briefly, then try it to the other side.

- *5–8-year-olds:* Allow the kids to move in and out of the pose from warrior 2 into this stretch. At the beginning ask them to stay in the pose for a few seconds, then build up to ten seconds.

- *8–11-year-olds:* Ask the children to stay in the posture for longer periods and focus on deep breathing. They can also begin to stretch their sides by slowly raising and lowering the upper hand – towards the ear and then down to the hip.

Warrior stretch lengthens the sides of the body and promotes trunk stability. It also encourages balance.

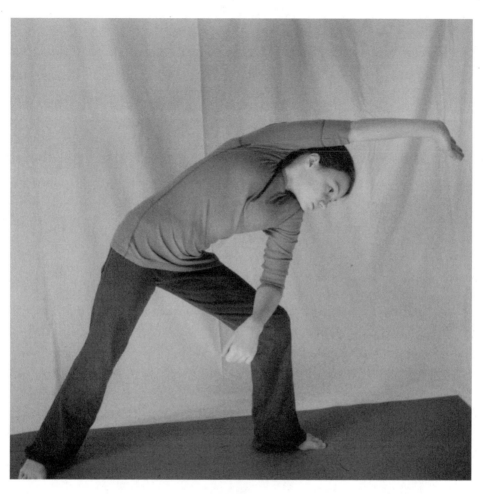

Warrior stretch

Triangle

Stand with feet just slightly wider than hip distance apart – right foot pointing out, the left slightly turned in. Breathe in and raise the arms up and out to the sides to shoulder level. Exhale and tip to the right side bringing the right hand to the right leg. Switch sides.

- *3–5-year-olds:* Have the kids move in and out of the pose, holding it briefly. Describe and look at triangles and objects made up of triangular shapes. Three kids can lay down on the floor to make a triangle. Use a digital camera to take a photo for immediate feedback.

- *5–8-year-olds:* Ask the children to move in and out of the posture before staying in pose. Have them point out objects or structures in the room that have angles.

- *8–11-year-olds:* Encourage the children to work through the practice several times and ask them to hold poses for longer periods. Experiment with looking up at the hand and down at the foot (this should be done slowly; it may cause dizziness in some children so exercise care). Begin discussing different kinds of angles.

Working through this practice stretches the torso.

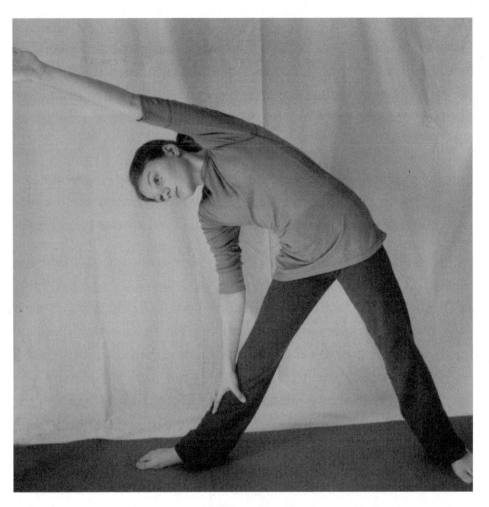

Triangle

Tree balance

Start in mountain pose. Lift the left foot up to the inside of the right leg (to the shin or to the thigh, depending on ability to balance – don't push on ankle or knee). Bring the hands together in front of the heart, then lift them straight overhead or stretch out diagonally like branches. Switch sides.

- *3–5-year-olds:* Let the kids move in and out of the posture as if they are trees blowing in a gentle wind. Have the children lay down on a large piece of paper and you trace around them in the pose. They can color or decorate the paper "trees".

- *5–8-year-olds:* Begin by staying in posture a little longer. Have the kids form a forest with their bodies, let them make wind sounds blowing through the trees. Discuss forests, trees, and wildlife. Complete the practice with an art activity that has a forest or tree theme. Perhaps the kids can work cooperatively to trace each other while laying on a large piece of paper in the pose. Kids with tactile sensitivity may be uncomfortable being traced; in which case they can be the "tracer" and then work with the other children to decorate the "tree".

- *8–11-year-olds:* Children of this age can maintain the pose for longer. Have them fix their gaze on a point in order to maintain balance. Experiment with what happens when they close their eyes.

Kids who have balance difficulties may attempt the pose near a wall or with an adult close to them so they can establish balance by holding on briefly, while you encourage them to use their own bodies to balance. Make sure the kids are breathing when attempting to balance, and remind them, as we often hold our breath when concentrating.

This pose helps promote balance, focus, and awareness.

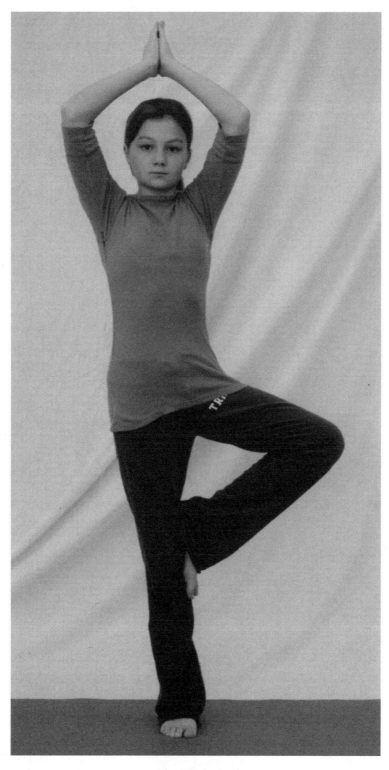

Tree balance

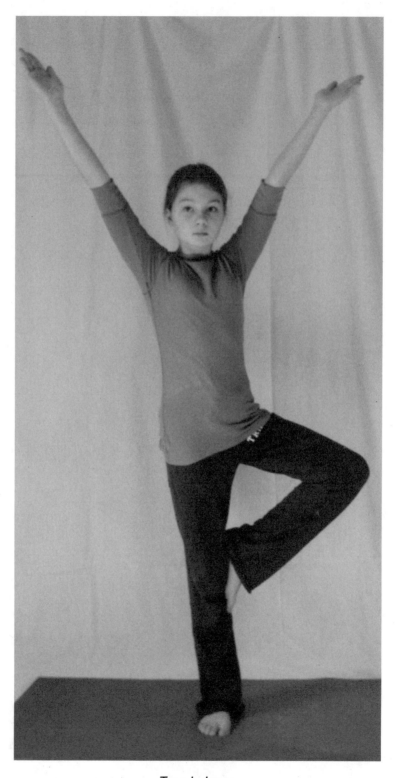

Tree balance

Dancer

Start in mountain pose. Bend the right leg at the knee and hold onto the top of the right foot. Breathe in and raise the left arm over the head. Breathe out and bend forward slightly from the hips, balancing on the left foot. Switch sides.

- *5–8-year-olds:* Encourage the kids to move in and out of the posture, then ask them to try holding the position. You can use soft music to help calm the children and exciting music for increased input. Don't use music with a fast tempo for balance postures; experiment with classical music selections. Following the practice, each child can then share a favorite dance move that the others can imitate, which will give all the kids a chance to be a leader. You could also incorporate the "freeze game" when the kids are showing their dance moves: the children dance to the music, you stop the music and the children must freeze in whatever position they are in. This is a good exercise through which to build strength and body awareness.

- *8–11-year-olds:* Children of this age can maintain the pose for longer. Tell them to find a point to fix their gaze upon in order to maintain balance. Experiment with what happens when they close their eyes. Kids who have balance difficulties can attempt the pose near a wall or with an adult close by so they can establish balance by holding on briefly. Do encourage them to use their bodies to balance. Make sure the kids are breathing when attempting to balance; remind them as needed.

This pose promotes balance, focus, and trunk stability.

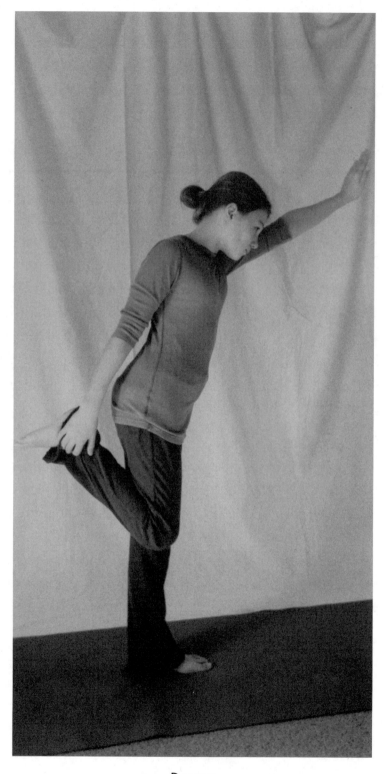

Dancer

Swinging twist

Stand with feet slightly wider than hip distance apart. Raise the arms to the sides at shoulder level. Swing the arms from one side to the other, rotating the trunk to increase the twist. Let the arms fly through the air during the twist.

- *3–5-year-olds:* Start slowly and increase the intensity, then have the children slow down again. For increased sensory input, put on *The Twist* song, or sing it yourself.

- *5–8-year-olds:* Experiment with the speed of the twisting – have them twist slow, then fast. Say "freeze" and the children have to stop in the middle of their movements and hold the pose like a statue until you tell them to continue to twist.

- *8–11-year-olds:* Start slowly then gradually twist with more intensity, then slow down until they come to a stop.

For increased input vary the speed and change the intensity. For a calming effect focus on a steady rhythm to the twisting, using a suitable piece of music to help.

The swinging twist encourages trunk rotation and provides vestibular input.

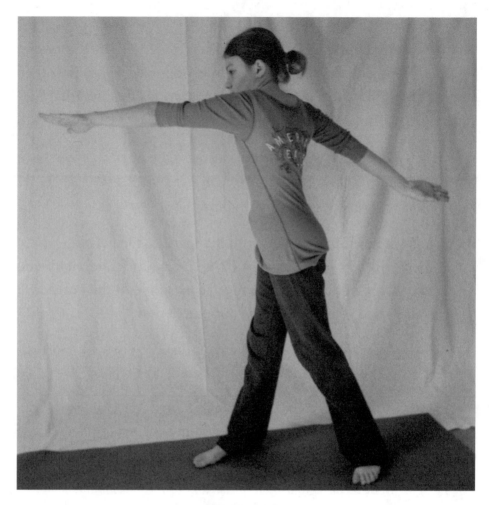

Swinging twist

Downward dog

This is a transitional posture which will be incorporated into the next chapter on sequencing. Begin on hands and knees, curl the toes under, breathe out and push up and backwards lifting the tailbone. Tuck the head under.

- *3–5-year-olds:* Encourage the kids to experiment with different kinds of barks, such as those that come from big dogs and those that come from small dogs. Whisper if the kids have auditory sensitivity or ask them to pretend to be silent well-behaved dogs.

- *5–8-year-olds:* Experiment with holding the posture and moving around in the posture. To get kids really excited play the song *Who Let the Dogs Out.* To calm them try a Disney animal- themed song.

- *8–11-year-olds:* Experiment with holding the posture for longer. Have the kids practice the breath of fire or belly breathing while in posture. The breath of fire should be used with kids who have under-responsive systems, while belly breathing or the langhana breath should be used for kids with hypersensitivities.

Performing this movement promotes proximal stability and shoulder and hip stability.

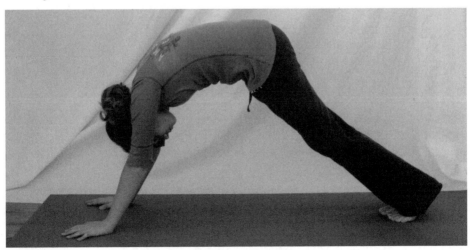

Downward dog

Dog to lunge

Begin in downward dog. Lift the right leg up and back, then swing the leg forward coming into a lunge. The head should be raised so that you are looking straight ahead. Push back into downward dog (lowering the head) and switch sides.

- *5–8-year-olds:* Move in and out of posture.

- *8–11-year-olds:* Move in and out of posture then ask the children to stay and hold the pose for a few practices. Staying in the pose will help build strength. The children should not be holding their breath. Remind them that they should be breathing throughout the practice.

Dog to lunge improves strength and stretches the legs.

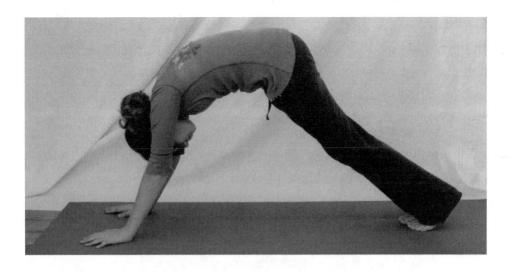

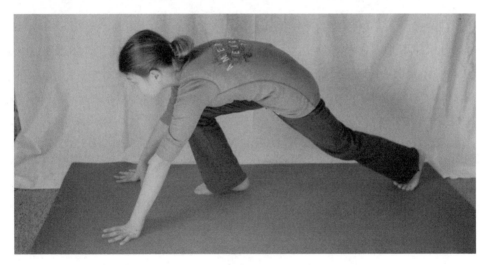

Dog to lunge

Camel

Begin in tall kneeling, with toes curled under. Breathe in, raise the arms over the head, exhale and reach behind grabbing the heels. Lift the belly and point the chin up to the ceiling.

- *5–8-year-olds:* Move in and out of position, holding the pose briefly. Incorporate fun discussions about camels; use photos and/or drawings. Have the kids draw their own camels.

- *8–11-year-olds:* Begin holding pose for a little longer. Initiate a discussion about camels, ask questions – where do camels live? what kinds of camels are there?

This pose will be difficult for kids with vestibular sensitivity. The post can be modified by reaching back to one ankle at a time. Kids who are under-responsive may enjoy the vestibular and proprioceptive intensity of camel. However, some kids can become easily overexcited by tipping their heads backwards. Be alert to this and proceed slowly. If the child does appear to be overexcited follow with a heavy weight-bearing pose such as plank.

Camel is a backbend that opens the front of the body. Children with low arousal and/or tone often slump which closes the front of the body. This is a great way to open them up. Camel is also an excitatory pose which can help kids when done prior to taking a test or quiz.

The camel opens and stretches the front of the body.

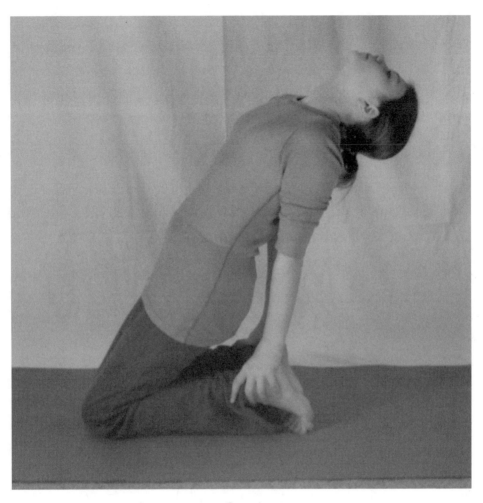

Camel

Gate

Begin in tall kneeling. Stretch one leg out to the side, with the foot on the floor. Raise the opposite arm straight up and place the other hand on the extended leg. Switch sides. Reach up and slightly bend sideways sliding the hand down the extended leg.

- *3–5-year-olds:* Assume pose briefly.

- *5–8-year-olds:* Experiment with holding the posture. Move in and out of the pose by bending the trunk into the pose, then straightening the trunk and lowering the arm.

- *8–11-year-olds:* Experiment with moving in and out of the pose, then stay in pose to build strength.

Practicing the gate stretches the sides of the body.

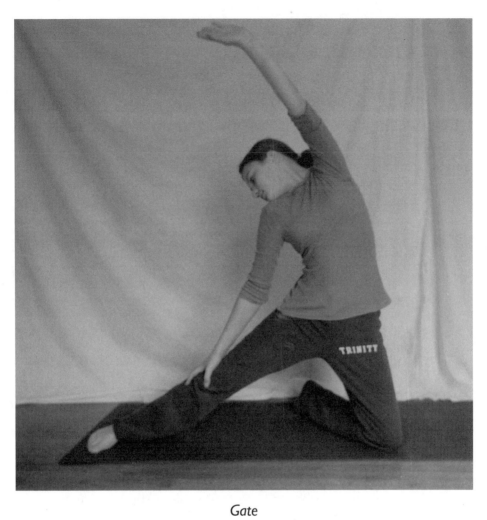

Gate

Cobra

Begin lying on the stomach with hands near the shoulders. Inhale and lift up, lifting the head, neck, and shoulders. Exhale to come down out of the pose. The hands are for stability, helping balance the upper body. Encourage the kids to lift the upper back, as this is an upper back strengthener.

- *3–5-year-olds:* Have the kids move in and out of cobra pose, make hissing sounds, and then move around the room on their bellies making sure they do not touch any of the other cobras. Color snake pictures. Talk about lines, and show straight and curved lines. Use long pieces of colored rope to make straight and curved lines.

- *5–8-year-olds:* Encourage the children to move in and out of the pose, and then stay in the pose. They can make hissing sounds and begin to move around the room on their bellies. Encourage discussion on snakes, and nature in general. Art projects, including drawing and coloring snakes, should be encouraged. If you have access to a play tunnel this would be a great time to use it. You can get knit interlock and have a cloth tunnel or use a standard tunnel. A cloth tunnel increases the tactile and deep pressure input.

- *8–11-year-olds:* Have the kids move in and out of pose, then ask them to stay in the pose. Make sure the children are breathing fully while maintaining the pose. A good follow-up activity can be related to snakes, nature, and science.

The cobra strengthens the upper back.

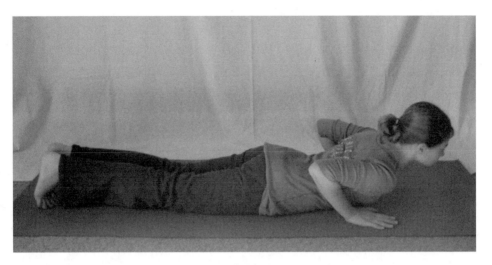

Cobra

Locust

Begin by lying on the stomach with arms extended in front of the body and palms of the hands on the floor. Raise opposite leg and arm, keeping both straight, slightly arching the back. Repeat to the other side.

- *3–5-year-olds:* Attempt pose briefly, to each side. Follow with an activity on a bug/insect theme.

- *5–8-year-olds:* Move in and out of pose, alternating to each side. Incorporate a discussion on bugs, including exoskeletons.

- *8–11-year-olds:* Move in and out of pose, alternating to each side. Begin to stay in pose on each side for brief periods to improve strength. Build in a science project related to insects and their importance in the food chain.

Locust promotes trunk stability and strength in the back of the body.

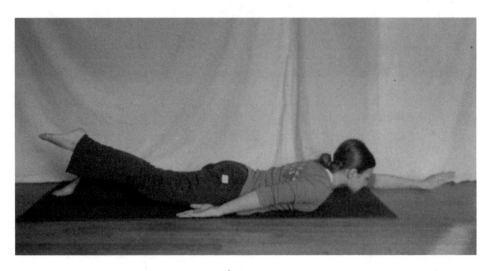

Locust

Bow

Begin by lying on the stomach. Bend the knees and reach back with the hands to grab the top of each foot. Pull the feet towards the body and lift the body up (legs and upper body).

- *3–5-year-olds:* Attempt pose briefly.

- *5–8-year-olds:* Move in and out of pose, then stay in pose. If the children are strong enough they can begin gentle rocking forwards and backwards.

- *8–11-year-olds:* Have the kids move in and out, and then stay in the pose. They can rock forwards and backwards, then side to side. Make sure that the children are not holding their breath. A follow-up activity could be a discussion on bows and arrows, and the types of cultures that used them.

Practicing this pose promotes body extension and strengthening.

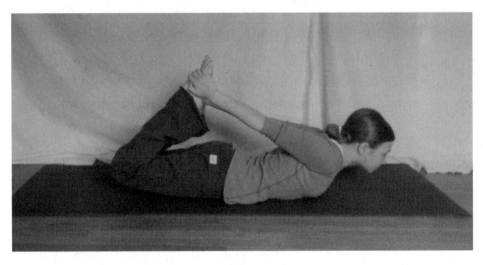

Bow

Stick pose

Sit with the legs straight out in front and arms at the sides of the body to help lift up the shoulders and upper back. Keep the back strong to sit up tall.

- *3–5-year-olds:* Have the kids assume stick pose and pretend they are rubbing all kinds of things onto their legs, arms, bellies, faces, and hair, with their hands. Some good pretend items are ketchup, mustard, peanut butter and jelly, mud or anything else fun the kids can think of. It's a good way to get some deep pressure onto their bodies.

- *5–8-year-olds:* Ask the children to assume stick pose and then let them experiment with different textures on their arms, legs, and face. You can use washcloths, bath brushes, paintbrushes, or anything else suitable you can think of. Compare soft versus scratchy. Go outside and look at and collect sticks. Use them as paintbrushes for an art project.

- *8–11-year-olds:* Move into stick pose and experiment with brushes (as above). You can also have the kids raise their arms over their heads and have them move just their bottoms to move forward and backward, rocking on each seat bone.

Kids with tactile sensitivity may be resistant to touch brushes; however, gentle coaxing and giving them time to try usually works, as long as they are in control of what is touching them.

The stick pose increases trunk strength and leg muscle lengthening.

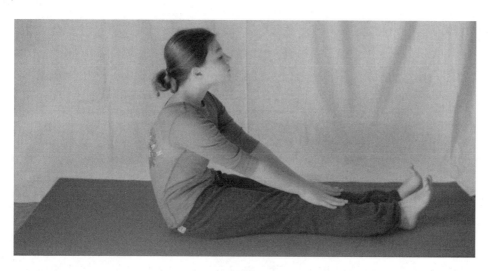

Stick pose

Boat

Sit with the knees bent up. Place the arms and hands around thighs, gently rock back and lift the legs and straighten the arms out in front.

- *3–5-year-olds:* Have the kids assume the posture but keep their arms and hands under their legs supporting themselves. They can begin gently rocking back and forth and discover their balance point. Talk about and experiment with things that float and sink.

- *5–8-year-olds:* The children rock back and forth balancing on their sitting bones. Then have them attempt the full posture with arms outstretched. Have a *Row your Boat* sing-along. Make charts and graphs of things that float and sink.

- *8–11-year-olds:* Let the kids assume the full posture. Have them sing-along as above or have them count out loud for as long as they can maintain the pose. Add a discussion on boats and draw pictures of boats on a lake or the ocean.

This posture promotes abdominal strength and balance.

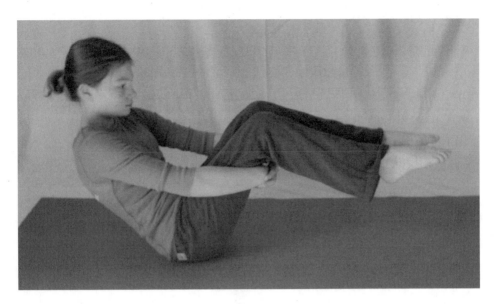

Boat

Twist

Sit with legs crossed. Breathe in and lift the body up, making it longer and taller. Exhale and twist by rotating the trunk, keeping both seat bones on the floor. If twisting to the right, the left hand can grasp the right knee to assist in the twist. The other hand can rest on the floor behind. After twisting the body, turn the head in the direction of the twist to look over the shoulder. Hold, then come back to center and repeat, twisting to the other side.

- *3–5-year-olds:* Have the children move gently in and out of posture, and then stay briefly.

- *5–8-year-olds:* Instruct the children to move in and out of posture then tell them to stay using a slow count of five to ten seconds on each side. Finish the activity with a pretzel snack. Some kids like a crunchy, salty snack – it helps them to focus. You can also discuss foods and taste preferences (salty, sweet, crunchy, etc.).

- *8–11-year-olds:* As above, but you could add the activity of making homemade pretzels. Measuring, mixing, and rolling dough are all good deep pressure activities. Snacking on a crunchy snack like pretzels can improve the attention and awareness level for some children.

The twist aids trunk rotation and stability.

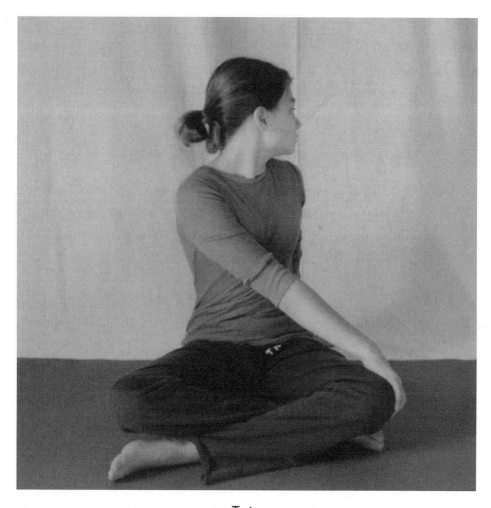

Twist

Tailor pose

Begin by sitting with the bottoms of the feet together and knees out. Slowly attempt to lower the knees to the floor. Once knees are lowered, gently bend forward at the hips and hold the feet.

- *3–5-year-olds:* Have the kids move slowly and gently in and out of posture, stay briefly, and sing a quiet song.

- *5–8-year-olds:* Instruct the children to move in and out of posture then stay for a short period; this could be a good time to sing a gentle song, or tell them a short story. Have the kids focus on their breathing and try to slow it down.

- *8–11-year-olds:* Have the kids move in and out of posture then stay for a longer period; this could be a good time to read a story. Encourage the children to focus on their breathing and try to slow it down. They can also try the breath of fire (if you are looking to increase alertness) or alternate nostril breathing (for calming).

This pose stretches the inner thighs.

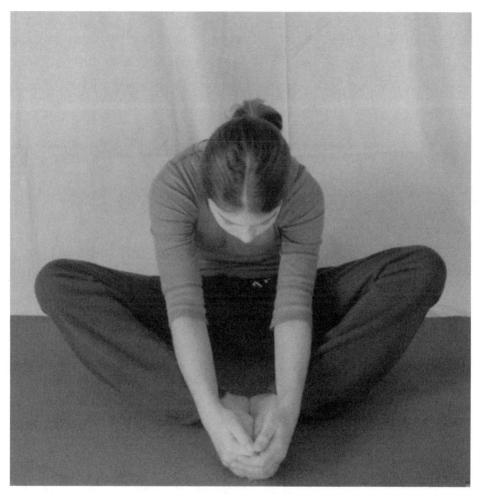

Tailor pose

Melting table

Begin on hands and knees with tips of toes on floor. Inhale and as you exhale lower and rock back until you are resting your bottom on your heels and your forehead is on the floor. As you come up inhale and then repeat.

- *3–5-year-olds:* Have the kids move slowly and gently in and out of posture. As a follow-up activity have a discussion with the children about different things that melt. Ask them what their favorite breakfast snack, lunch or dinner is while they are in the table pose.

- *5–8-year-olds:* Instruct the children to move in and out of posture. Experiment with the speed of the movement – first go really slow, then increase the speed until they are doing it quickly, then slow down until they are moving in slow motion.

- *8–11-year-olds:* Children of this age can use this pose as a warm up or cool down. Experiment with the speed of the movement as above.

Practicing the melting table promotes spine movement.

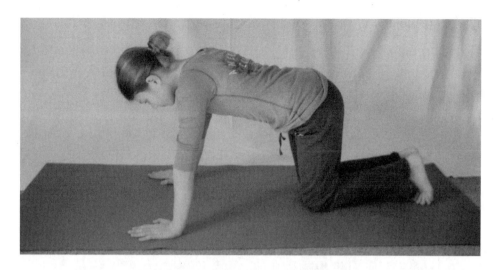

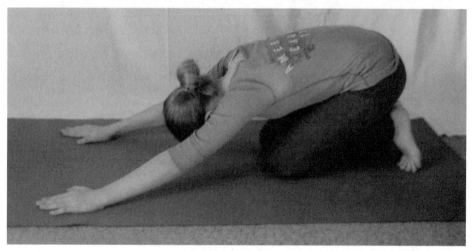

Melting table

Cat stretching

Begin on hands and knees, with tips of toes on the floor. Inhale and lift the left leg out behind you as you lift the right arm out in front of you. Exhale while lowering the arm and leg. Switch sides.

- *3–5-year-olds:* Have the kids move in and out of the posture, while meowing and purring. Ask them if they have a pet, or if they were a cat what would their name be?

- *5–8-year-olds:* Move in and out of posture then begin to hold the balance pose with arm and leg lifted. Kids can meow or purr. Discuss the qualities of a cat (soft, gentle, curious etc).

- *8–11-year-olds:* Instruct the children to practice the posture and then begin to challenge their balance by staying in the posture for longer periods. Discuss pets and why we love them, what is important about our pets, etc. Begin discussing compassion and why we should treat animals with compassion and respect. Some kids who under-register sensory input (tactile and proprioceptive) often handle pets roughly, without realizing that they are squeezing them too hard. It is a good opportunity to talk about being gentle and grading the touch.

This stretch improves trunk strength and balance.

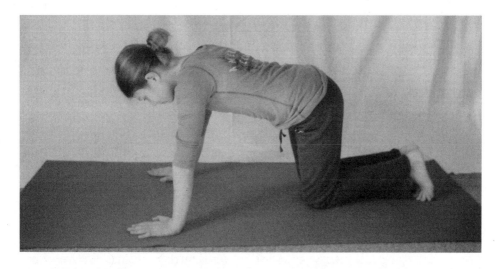

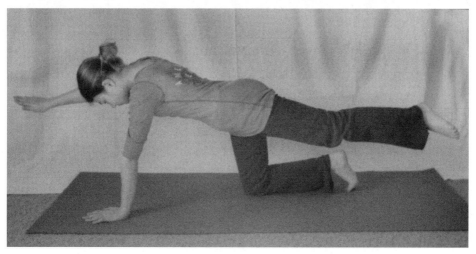

Cat stretching

Walking plank

Begin on hands and knees with tips of toes on the floor. Walk the feet out behind you and hold in a push-up position. (You should be bearing your weight on your hands and the balls of your feet.) Walk forwards, backwards, and sideways.

- *3–5-year-olds:* The children should briefly maintain pose, then rest.

- *5–8-year-olds:* Have the kids assume pose and then begin to move around by walking forwards and backwards; they can pretend they are alligators, crocodiles, or lizards. Discuss where these animals live and what they eat.

- *8–11 year-olds:* Assume the posture for longer periods and begin to move in all directions. The kids can pretend they are alligators, crocodiles, lizards, kimono dragons – whatever they want. Discuss where these animals live, what they eat, if they are in danger of becoming extinct. Paint, color, or draw pictures of the animals.

This is a good counter-pose for children who seem to become overstimulated in some of the other poses, because it allows weight bearing in the arms and feet.

This pose promotes strength and proximal stability.

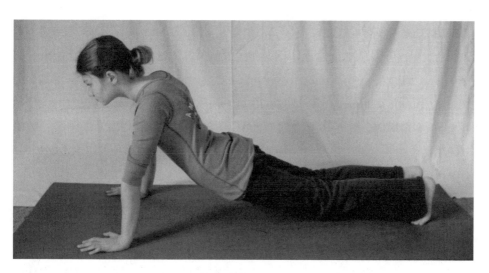

Walking plank

Upside down kid[**]

Start sitting with knees bent in front. Rock backwards and roll through until the body is supported by the back of the shoulders. Lift legs up to the sky, placing the hands on the lower back for support. Be sure that the kids are supported on their shoulders, not on their necks. Children with breathing difficulties or any neck contraindications should not assume this posture.

- *5–8-year-olds:* Have the kids assume posture and stay for several breaths, coming in and out of posture as needed.

- *8–11-year-olds:* Children of this age can begin to stay in posture for longer periods; have them practice belly breathing.

This is a difficult posture for kids with vestibular sensitivities; begin by having them put their legs up on a wall. Some children may become overexcited in this pose, and it can manifest by acting out or becoming extremely silly. If this happens, follow with a pose such as walking plank or try to relax them and focus on slow breathing.

Practicing this posture promotes relaxation.

[**]   Children with Down Syndrome can have instability in the first and second vertebrae and should have a physician's approval prior to attempting this pose.

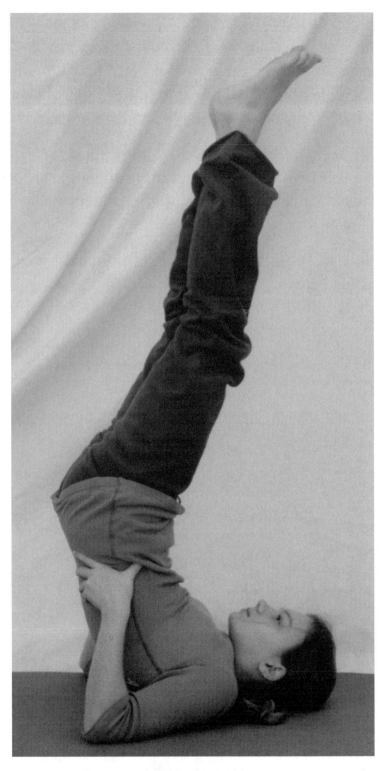

Upside down kid

Crow

Squat down and place the hands between the feet. Rest the inside of your legs on the outside of your arms. Begin to bend forward, placing your weight onto your hands and lifting your feet off of the floor as you balance.

- *5–8-year-olds:* Have the kids move in and out of posture, then begin to hold briefly. This is a good opportunity to discuss different kinds of birds, make bird feeders, and draw and color pictures of birds.

- *8–11-year-olds:* Encourage the children to balance in pose for longer periods. All of the follow-up activities suggested above would be suitable; in addition you could work on a science project related to balance and weight distribution.

The crow pose develops arm strength, balance, and mental focus.

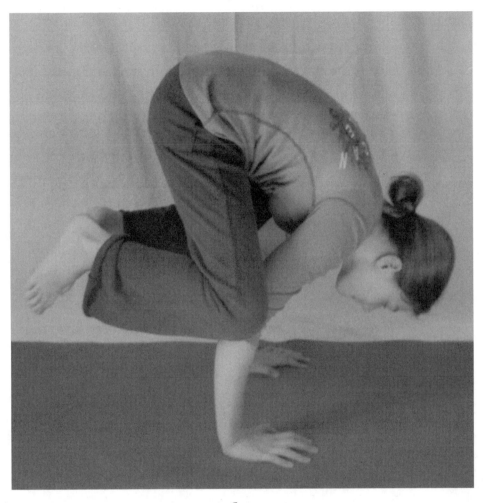

Crow

Rag doll

Lie face-up on the floor. Close the eyes and turn hands palm upwards.
Tense the body and squeeze all the muscles, from the head to the feet.
Let go and relax completely.

- *All ages:* relaxation is important for children of all ages. Have the
  kids tense and release their muscles to feel the difference between
  tension and relaxation. Explain tension and relaxation to them.
  Allow the kids to maintain the pose; older children will be able
  to hold the posture for longer. Use relaxation music or a meditation and guided imagery on a beautiful and relaxing place. Describe the place as the most peaceful place on earth. This can be a
  place they can visualize when they are under stress.

This pose is relaxing and helps the children distinguish muscle tension from muscle relaxation.

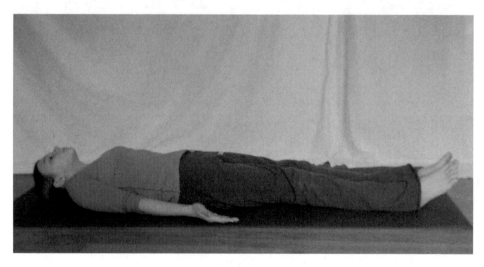

Rag doll

Sequencing poses

Moving through a series of poses allows the development of concentration and strength.

The sun salute

The sun salute is a series of poses designed to create heat in the body. It is important to use breath and movement. The sequence can be performed slowly, moving with soft, grounding, background music for kids who need centering, or quicken the pace and use music with a faster rhythm to get the kids going.

The series of postures is as follows:

Begin in *mountain* pose, exhale to *fold in half*, step back to *walking plank*; lower down on the exhale, inhale into *cobra*, exhale and push back into *downward dog*; inhale into *dog to lunge*, exhale, stepping forward into *fold in half* and inhale into *mountain*.

Begin with the right foot forward into a lunge, and then repeat the whole sequence starting with the left foot. This series can be repeated over and over.

- This sequence is best for the 5–8-year-old and 8–11-year-old age groups.

Center follow-up activities on the subject of the sun – discussions, art projects etc. Broaden the theme to include planets and the solar system.

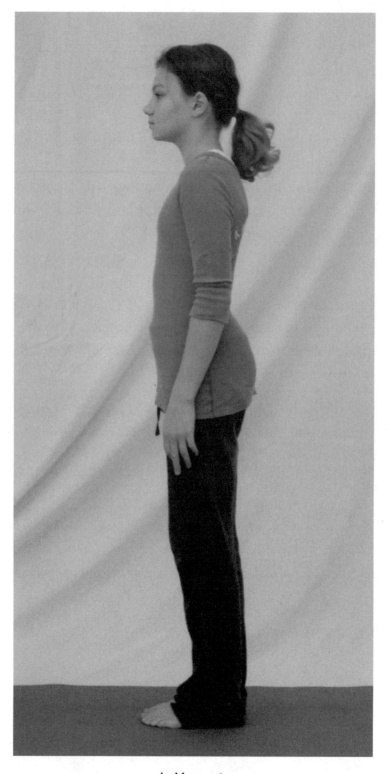

1. Mountain

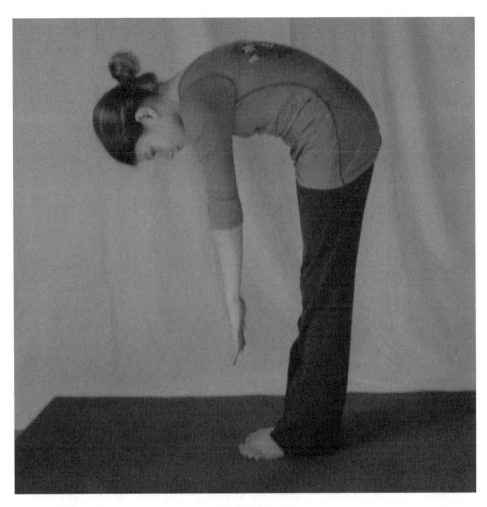

2. Fold in half

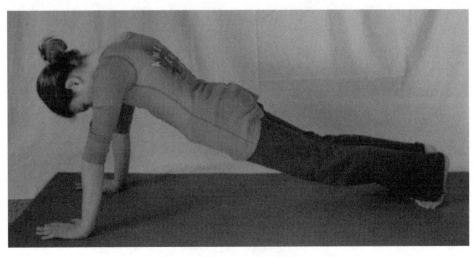

3. Walking plank

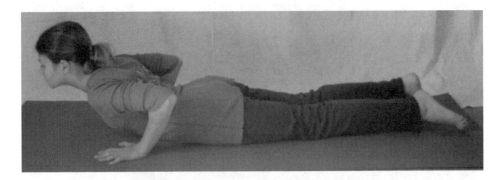

4. Cobra

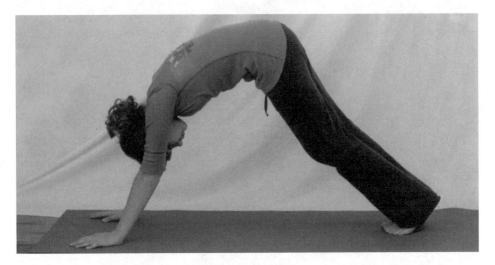

5. Downward dog

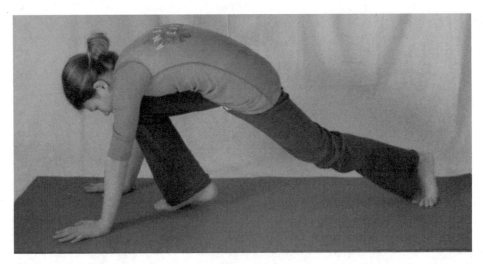

6. Dog to lunge

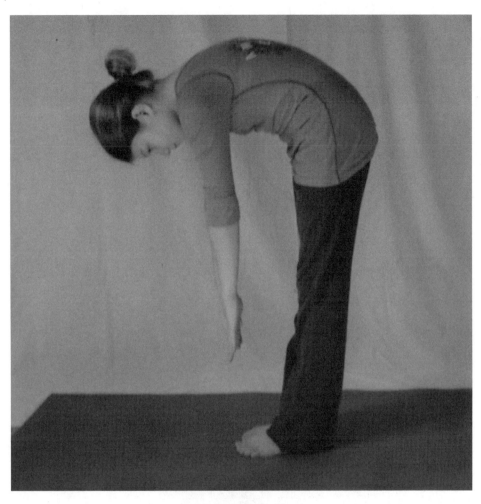

7. Fold in half

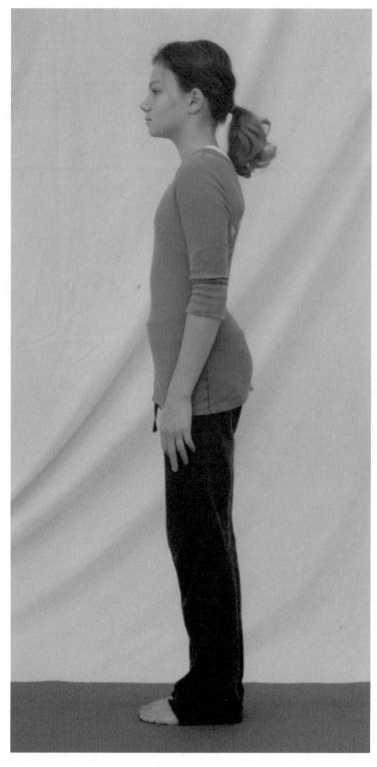

8. Mountain

The moon salute

A series of poses designed to have the cooling and calming qualities of
the moon. The sequence can be performed slowly, accompanied by slow
grounding music for kids who need centering, or the pace quickened
using music with a faster beat to stimulate the children.

The series of postures is as follows:

Begin in *melting table*, inhale into *cat stretch*, exhale into *melting table*; from
hands and knees exhale into *downward dog*, inhale into *dog to lunge*, drop
the back knee to the floor, then bring the knees to meet and come into a
tall kneeling position; curl the toes under and come into *camel*, then back
into *melting table*.

Start with the right foot forward into a lunge, and then repeat the whole
sequence beginning with the left foot. This series can be repeated over
and over. The moon salute is best for the 5–8-year-old and 8–11-year
-old age groups.

Follow-up activities can be art projects and discussions about the moon.
Take the opportunity to discuss planets and the solar system.

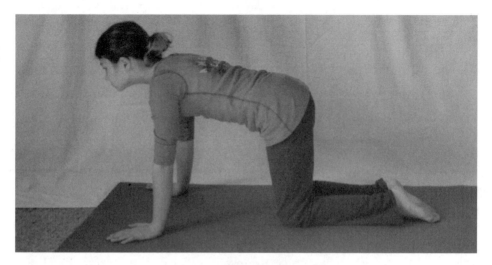

1. Melting table

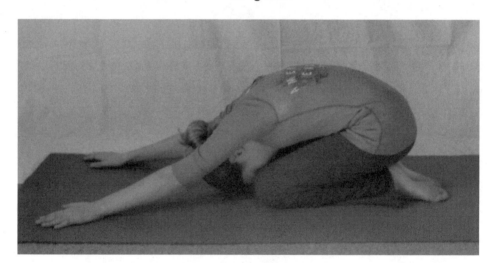

2. Melting table

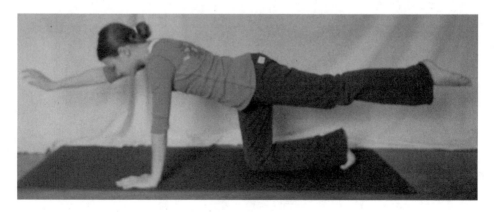

3. Cat stretch

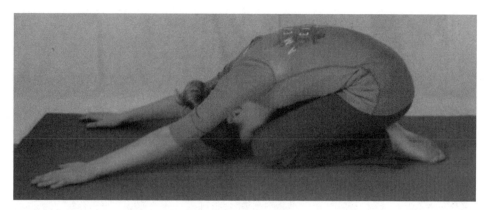

4. Melting table

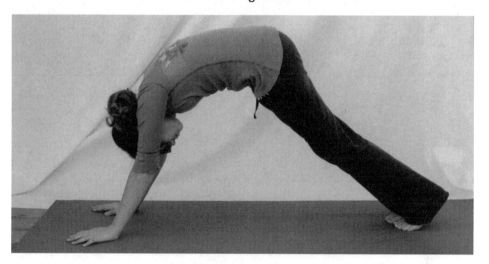

5. Downward dog

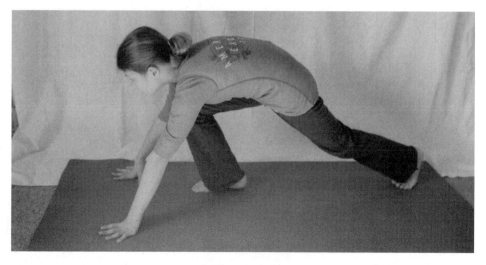

6. Dog to lunge

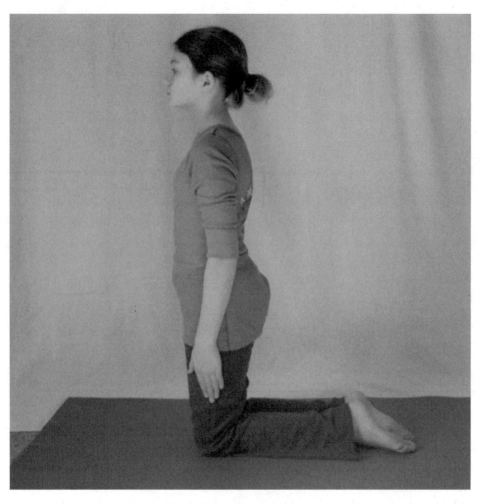

7. *Tall kneeling position*

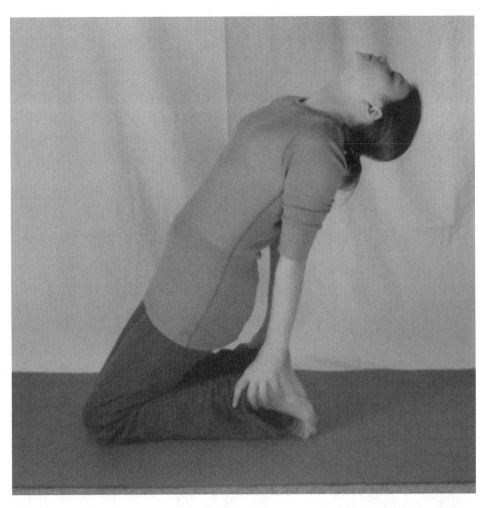

8. Camel

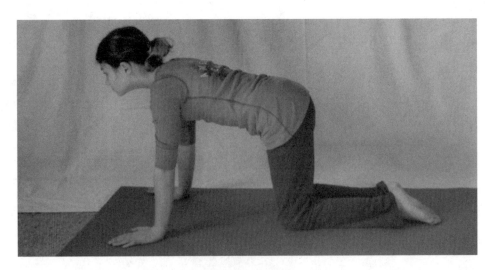

9. Melting table

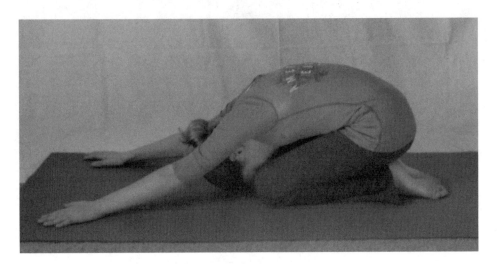

10. Melting table

Suggested Reading

Ayres, J.A. (1979) *Sensory Integration and the Child.* Los Angeles: Western Psychological Services.

Dennison, P.E. and Dennison, G.E. (1994) *Brain Gym, Simple Activities for Whole Brain Learning.* Ventura, CA: Edu-Kinesthetics.

Desikachar, T.K.V. (1980) *Religiousness in Yoga.* New York: University Press of America.

Iyengar, B.K.S. (1966) *Light on Yoga.* New York: Schocken Books.

Kraftsow, G. (1999) *Yoga for Wellness.* New York: Penguin Compass.

List of Poses

Index

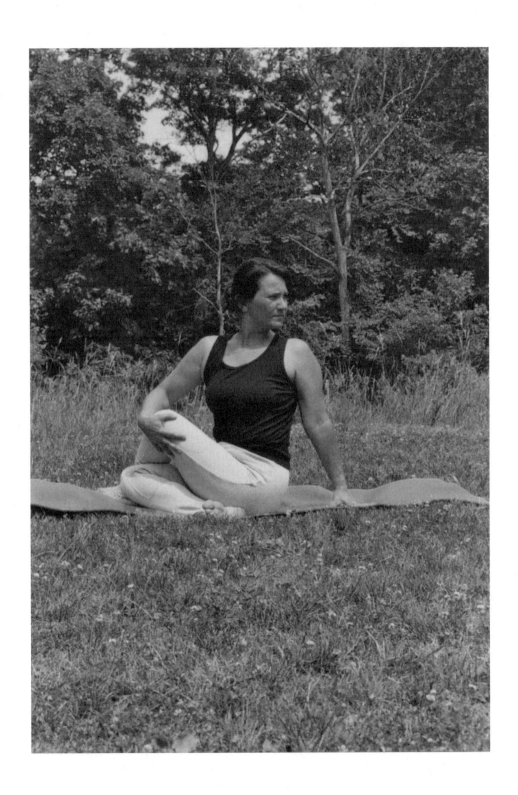